Freestyle 2018:

The Essential Freestyle Guide to Rapid Weight Loss for Beginners - Includes Delicious Easy Recipes For Melting The Fat Away Quickly & Effectively

Table of Contents

Introduction

It is an undisputed fact that countless people around the world are suffering from a string of health problems and issues. Much of it can be attributed to lifestyle choices, and a huge part comes down to the food that they consume. While there are plenty of diets and fads out there promoted with the aim to help people get rid of their health and fitness problems, much of them either limit or restrict what you can or cannot eat, which makes the dieting process for many people miserable and not the least motivating whatsoever.

However, this doesn't have to be the case with this freestyle program as it not only simple in its follow through, but it gives you the freedom to still enjoy your dishes and the meals you'd like to eat.

What you are about to learn inside this book are all sorts of recipes that you can cook and enjoy for breakfast, lunch, dinner, and will help you hit your goals this year to lose weight, melt the fat away and live the lifestyle you desire.

Say goodbye to diets and fads that don't work and let's get straight into the book!

Breakfast

Tasty Blueberry and Corn Pancakes

COOKING TIME: 10 minutes

SERVES: 8

INGREDIENTS:

- 2 cups all-purpose flour,
- ½ cup yellow cornmeal,
- ¼ teaspoon salt,
- 1 ¾ cups low-fat (1%) milk,
- ½ cup fat-free egg substitute,
- 2 tablespoons sugar,
- 1 tablespoon plus 1 teaspoon baking powder,
- 1 tablespoon canola oil,
- ¾ cup fresh corn kernels or frozen corn kernels
- 6 tablespoons pure maple syrup (warmed)

INSTRUCTIONS:

1) Thoroughly mix together flour, cornmeal, sugar, baking powder, and salt in a medium bowl.

2) Combine the milk, egg substitute, and oil in a well situated in the center of the flour mixture; with a fork stir until mixed thoroughly.

3) With a rubber spatula, stir flour mixture into the milk mixture just until flour mixture is moistened. Gently stir in blueberries and corn.

4) Spray a griddle with nonstick spray and set over medium heat. Pour a ¼ cup of batter onto the griddle. Cook until bubbles appear and edges of pancakes look dry about 4 minutes.

5) Turn pancakes over and cook until golden brown on the second side, about 3 minutes longer. Transfer to a platter and keep warm. Repeat with remaining batter, once done. Serve with maple syrup.

Delicious Freestyle Pimento Chile Chicken

Ingredients:

- 2 ½ c. cooked, chopped chicken breast (chopped into about 1/2" cubes
- ½ c. fat free chicken broth
- 1 ½ c. 98% fat free cream of mushroom soup (I use Campbell's)
- 1 ½ c. Healthy Request Condensed cream of chicken soup
- 1 4-oz. jar pimentos, drained (1/2 c.)
- 2 4-oz. cans Hatch green chiles, chopped and drained (You can add a 3rd can if you're just crazy about chiles like I am.)
- 10 oz. 50% reduced fat sharp cheddar cheese
- 6 oz. of Doritos (by weight) toasted corn tortilla chips, slightly crushed
- Pickled jalapeños, green onions, and/or cherry tomatoes for serving (optional)

Instructions:

1. Mix all ingredients except Doritos and cheese. In a large casserole dish (I use 9" x 13"), layer ½ of chicken mixture, then ½ of cheese, then ½ of the Doritos.
2. Repeat the same layers once more, ending with Doritos on top. Bake at 350° for about 40-45 minutes.

3. Cover top with foil if Doritos begin to brown too much. Serve with pickled jalapeños and/or your favorite salsa.

Heavenly Roast Pork With Ginger and Green Beans

COOKING TIME: 35 minutes

SERVES: 2

INGREDIENTS:

2 tablespoons minced peeled fresh ginger,

1 tablespoon reduced-sodium soy sauce,

1 tablespoon dry sherry,

1 tablespoon hoisin sauce,

1 teaspoon chili-garlic sauce,

1 teaspoon dark sesame oil,

1 (1lb.) trimmed pork tenderloin,

¾ lb. trimmed green beans,

6-scallions (cut crosswise in half)

INSTRUCTIONS:

1) Preheat oven to 425F. Spray a large heavy roasting pan with nonstick spray.

2) Whisk together the ginger, soy sauce, sherry, hoisin sauce, chili-garlic sauce, and oil in small bowl until mixed well. Toss together the beans, scallions, and remaining ginger mixture in a large bowl.

3) Place pork to one side of prepared pan. Place beans on other side of the pan. Roast until instant-read thermometer inserted

into the center of pork registers 145F for medium and beans are very tender, about 25 minutes.

4) Transfer pork to cutting board and let stand 10 minutes. Cut pork across grain into 12 slices and serve with beans.

Serve and enjoy.

Tasty Slow Cooker Chili

COOKING TIME: 4-5 hours

SERVES: 6

INGREDIENTS:

½ pound extra lean ground beef or turkey,

1 medium green bell pepper (deseeded, diced),

1 medium red bell pepper(deseeded, diced),

1 teaspoon garlic(minced),

14 ounces canned crushed tomatoes,

2 tablespoons canned diced green chilies or 1 small jalapeño pepper (sliced),

7.5 ounces canned kidney beans (drained, rinsed),

1 teaspoon ground cumin,

1 tablespoon chili powder,

1 small onion(chopped),

Salt to taste,

Pepper to taste

and 1 tablespoon tomato paste

INSTRUCTIONS:

1) Place a skillet over medium heat. Add beef and garlic and sauté until brown. Break it simultaneously as it cooks. Add bell

peppers and sauté for a couple of minutes. Add cumin and chili powder and stir.

2) Transfer into the slow cooker. Add rest of the ingredients and stir well.

3) Cover and cook on 'High' for 4-5 hours. Ladle into bowls and serve.

Delicious Mustard & Baked Beans

Ready in 1 hr.

4 servings

Ingredients:

- 1 lb. small white beans
- 1 small onion, diced
- 2 minced cloves garlic
- ½ cup molasses
- ½ cup maple syrup
- 1 tablespoon mustard powder
- ½ cup vinegar
- Ground pepper
- 4-6 cups of water
- 2 teaspoon salt

Instructions:

1. Soak beans overnight with cold water. Discard and rinse the beans and over with 5 cups of fresh water.

Cook the beans with the "Bean/Chili" setting at high pressure for 10 minutes until they start softening.

2. Skim and discard any frothy stuff. Add the rest of the ingredients, top up water and pressure cook on "bean" setting for about 45 minutes until the beans soften

Nutrition information

Calories: 392

Carbohydrates: 55g

Fats: 13g

Proteins: 14g

Yummy Cinnamon Rolls

Ingredients:

¼ c. cream cheese

¼ c. sugar

¼ tsp. vanilla

1 tsp. butter, melted

11 oz. breadstick dough, cold

2 Tbsp. brown sugar

1 tsp. cinnamon

Directions:

1. Turn on the oven and let it heat up to 375 degrees. While that is heating up, take out a baking pan and prepare it with some cooking spray.

2. Take out a small bowl and mix together the brown sugar, cinnamon, and the butter and place to the side.

3. Take the breadstick dough and make it into 12 strips. Sprinkle on some brown sugar to this dough and then roll them into a spiral. Press the dough down to seal up the ends.

4. Place these rolls into a baking pan, leaving them about an inch apart. Place into the oven and let them

bake for 15 minutes. When they are done, take out of the oven and let them cool for 10 minutes.

5. While the rolls are baking, work on the frosting. Bring out a bowl and mix together the cream cheese, sugar, and vanilla. Add a bit of water to this until you get the consistency that you would like.

6. Drizzle this frosting onto the prepared rolls and let it set for a few minutes before serving.

Mouth Watering Spaghetti Squash in the Pot

Ready in 12- 15 minutes

4 servings

Ingredients

- 1 spaghetti squash
- 2 cups water

Instructions

1. Slice spaghetti squash along the length and remove the seeds.
2. Add 1 cup of water to the instant pot.
3. Stack the squash on top of each other with the cut-side up.
4. Tightly close the pot using the lid.
5. Bring heat to maximum with high-pressure for 5 minutes.
6. Release steam by turning the turning the vent on the top of the lid.
7. Allow 5 minutes for the pressure and steam to dissipate.

8. Open the lid and use a fork to test whether the spaghetti squash has been cooked.

Nutrition information

Calories: 31

Carbohydrates: 7g

Fats: 0.6g

Proteins: 0.6g

Scrumptious Rice & Mushroom Risotto

Ready in 30 minutes,

5-6 servings

Ingredients

- 1/2 cup white onion, minced
- 4 cloves minced garlic
- 1 tablespoon olive oil
- 5 ounces' mushrooms, chopped into small pieces
- salt and thyme, 1 teaspoon each
- 3 cups vegetable broth
- 1 cup dry white wine
- 2 cups Arborio rice
- 1/2 cup lemon juice
- 3 cups fresh spinach
- 1 tablespoon vegan butter substitute
- 1 tablespoon nutritional yeast
- Black pepper

Instructions

1. Turn rice cooker and leave the lid open. Add the oil and let it heat.

2. Add the onions and garlic, stir gently to soften. Stir in the mushrooms, thyme and salt.

3. Add the wine and vegetable broth, stir continuously.

4. Add Arborio rice and stir well.

5. Cover the cooker tightly with lid and restart the cooking timer.

6. Allow rice cook as per the prescribed cycle, stir well when cooking is complete.

7. Transfer rice into a serving bowl. Stir in lemon juice, vegan butter substitute, spinach, nutritional yeast and black pepper until the butter substitute melts completely and all the rest of ingredients are well stirred together. Serve warm.

Nutrition information
Calories: 454.5
Carbohydrates: 36.4g
Fats: 15.2g
Proteins: 0g

Mouth Watering Freestyle Greek Chickpea Salad Nutrition Information

Serves: 8 servings,

Serving size: ½ cup,

Calories: 192

Fat: 4 g,

Saturated fat: 1 g,

Trans fat: 0 g

Carbohydrates: 32 g,

Sugar: 6 g,

Sodium: 1297 mg

Fiber: 8 g,

Protein: 10 g,

Cholesterol: 4 mg

INGREDIENTS

- 2 (15 ounce) cans chickpea, drained and rinsed
- 1 small tomato, chopped
- ¼ cup finely chopped red onion
- ½ teaspoon sugar
- ¼ cup reduced fat crumbled feta cheese
- ½ tablespoon lemon juice
- ½ tablespoon red wine vinegar
- 1 tablespoon plain nonfat Greek Yogurt
- 2 cloves garlic, minced
- ¼ teaspoon salt
- ¼ teaspoon pepper
- 1-2 tablespoons cilantro

INSTRUCTIONS

1. Drain and rinse the chickpeas and place in a medium bowl.
2. Toss in the rest of the ingredients until chickpeas are evenly coated and all of the ingredients are mixed well.
3. Serve immediately and refrigerate any leftovers.

Heavenly Freestyle One Pot Garlicky Cuban Pork

213 calories

TOTAL TIME: 80 minutes plus marinade time

INGREDIENTS:

- 3 lb. boneless pork shoulder blade roast, lean, all fat removed
- 6 cloves garlic
- juice of 1 grapefruit (about 2/3 cup)
- juice of 1 lime
- 1/2 tablespoon fresh oregano
- 1/2 tablespoon cumin
- 1 tablespoon kosher salt
- 1 bay leaf
- lime wedges, for serving
- chopped cilantro, for serving
- hot sauce, for serving
- tortillas, optional for serving
- salsa, optional for serving

DIRECTIONS:

PRESSURE COOKER:

1. Cut the pork in 4 pieces and place in a bowl.

2. In a small blender or mini food processor, combine garlic, grapefruit juice, lime juice, oregano, cumin and salt and blend until smooth.

3. Pour the marinade over the pork and let it sit room temperature 1 hour or refrigerated as long as overnight.

4. Transfer to the pressure cooker, add the bay leaf, cover and cook high pressure 80 minutes. Let the pressure release naturally.

5. Remove pork and shred using two forks.

6. Remove liquid from pressure cooker, reserving then place the pork back into pressure cooker. Add about 1 cup of the liquid (jus) back, adjust the salt as needed and keep warm until you're ready to eat.

SLOW COOKER:

1. Cut the pork in 4 pieces and place in a bowl.

2. In a small blender or mini food processor, combine garlic, grapefruit juice, lime juice, oregano, cumin and salt and blend until smooth.

3. Pour the marinade over the pork and let it sit room temperature 1 hour or refrigerated as long as overnight.

4. Transfer to the slow cooker, add the bay leaf, cover and cook low 8 hours.

5. Remove pork and shred using two forks.

6. Remove liquid from slow cooker, reserving then place the pork back into slow cooker. Add about 1 cup of the liquid (jus) back, adjust the salt as needed and keep warm until you're ready to eat.

NUTRITION INFORMATION

Yield: 10 servings,

Serving Size: a little over 3 oz.

Amount Per Serving:

- Calories: 213
- Total Fat: 9.5g
- Saturated Fat: 0g
- Cholesterol: 91mg

- Sodium: 440.5mg
- Carbohydrates: 2.5g
- Fiber: 0.5g
- Sugar: 1.5g
- Protein: 26.5g

Irresistible Freestyle Ham & Apricot Dijon Glaze

145 calories

TOTAL TIME: 5 hours

INGREDIENTS:

- 1 (6 to 7 pound) Hickory smoked fully cooked spiral cut ham
- 5 tbsp. apricot preserves
- 2 tablespoons Dijon mustard

DIRECTIONS:

1. Make the glaze: Whisk 4 tablespoons of preserves and mustard together.
2. Place the ham in a 6-quart or larger slow cooker, making sure you can put the lid on. You may have to turn the ham on its side if your ham is too large.
3. Brush the glaze over the ham. Cover and cook on the LOW setting for 4 to 5 hours. Brush the remaining tablespoon of preserves over the ham the 30 minutes.

NUTRITION INFORMATION
Yield: 16,

Serving Size: 3 ounces

- Amount Per Serving:
- Smart Points: 5
- Points +: 5
- Calories: 145
- Total Fat: 7g
- Saturated Fat: 1.5g
- Sodium: 851mg
- Carbohydrates: 12g
- Fiber: 0g
- Sugar: 11g
- Protein: 15g

Delicious Tomato Spinach Soup

COOKING TIME: 4 hours

SERVES: 4

INGREDIENTS:

1 medium carrot(chopped),

5 ounces baby spinach,

1 medium stalk celery(chopped),

1 clove garlic(minced),

1 medium onion(chopped),

2 cups vegetable broth,

Salt to taste,

Pepper to taste,

½ teaspoon dried oregano

½ tablespoon dried basil,

¼ teaspoon crushed red pepper flakes,

14 ounces canned diced tomatoes

and 1 bay leaf

INSTRUCTIONS:

1) Add all the ingredients into the slow cooker. Clover and set on High for 5 hours.

2) Discard bay leaf and stir. Ladle into soup bowls and serve

Heavenly Freestyle BBQ Apricot Chicken

Prep time: 5 mins,

Cook time: 30 mins,

Total time: 35m

Serves: 6

Ingredients

- 1-pound boneless skinless chicken breasts
- ½ cup sugar-free apricot jam
- ½ cup G Hughes Sugar Free BBQ Sauce
- 2 tablespoons low sodium soy sauce
- 1 teaspoon garlic powder
- 1 teaspoon onion powder
- 1 teaspoon ground ginger

Instructions

1. In a medium bowl, whisk together the jam, bbq sauce, soy sauce, and seasonings.
2. Line baking sheet with foil and place chicken breasts in even layer
3. Pour barbecue sauce over chicken making sure well covered.
4. Bake at 350 degrees for 30 minutes.
5. Remove from oven, and serve with favorite sides.

Mouth Watering Healthy Morning Cookies

Ingredients:

2 egg whites

1/3 c. unsweetened cocoa

1/3 c. chocolate chips, mini

½ c. brown sugar, pressed down

½ c. sugar

1/8 tsp. salt

¼ c. butter, softened

1 c. flour

¼ tsp. baking soda

Directions:

1. Turn on the oven and let it heat up to 350 degrees. Take out a cookie sheet and spray it with some cooking spray.

2. Now take out a bowl and mix together the baking soda, flour, and salt. In a second bowl, combine the butter and the brown sugar and mix together until fluffy.

3. Add in the sugar to this second bowl and continue to beat to make it well incorporated. Put all of this into

the flour mixture and keep on stirring to combine. Now add in the chocolate chips.

4. Place small amounts of this onto the cookie sheet and then put into the oven and let it bake for about 10 minutes.

5. Take out of the oven and allow the cookies to cool down for a few minutes before taking them off the pan and cooling down completely.

Heavenly Apple Cinnamon Crisp

COOKING TIME: 8minutes

SERVES: 10

INGREDIENTS:

3/4 cup rolled oats,

1/2 cup water,

1/2 tsp nutmeg,

2 tsp cinnamon,

1/4 cup brown sugar,

1/4 cup flour,

4 tbsp butter,

1 tbsp maple syrup,

4 medium apples (peeled and chopped)

and 1/2 tsp salt

INSTRUCTIONS:

1) Place chopped apples on the bottom of the instant pot.

2) Sprinkle with nutmeg and cinnamon. Add maple syrup and water. Mix well.

3) Melt butter in a bowl and mix together melted butter, brown sugar, salt, oats, and flour. Add spoonful on top of apple mixture.

4) Seal instant pot with lid. Select manual high pressure for 8 minutes.

5) Use natural release method to open the instant pot.

Serve warm with vanilla ice-cream and enjoy.

Delicious Pressure Cooker Steamed Rice

Ready in 25 minutes,

4 servings.

Ingredients

- 1 cup Basmati or any long grain white rice

- 2 cups water

- 1 teaspoon olive oil

Instructions

1. Add the rice, water and oil to the pressure cooker. Cover cooker with lid.

2. Cook in high heat and high pressure. Lower the heat, maintain it and cook for up to 4 minutes.

3. Open the cooker with the natural release method. Transfer the cooker from the burner without removing the lid.

4. Instead, allow 10 minutes for the contents completely cook and steam. Fluff with a fork and serve.

Nutrition information

Calories: 199

Carbohydrates: 44.7g

Fats: 0.4g

Proteins: 4.2g

Irresistible Bean Soup

12 approximately 1 cup servings

Ingredients:

- 2 cans white beans (rinsed and drained)
- 2 cans Lima beans (rinsed and drained)
- 2 cans corn kernels drained
- 1 carton low sodium vegetable broth
- 12 slices Canadian Bacon chopped into small pieces
- Season to taste,

Directions:

1. Dump all ingredients into a large crockpot.
2. Stir gently to evenly mix ingredients.
3. Cook on low 6-8 hours.

Tasty Freestyle Butter Chicken Pot Pasta

Yield: 8 (1 1/4 CUPS) SERVINGS

INGREDIENTS:

- 1 ½ lbs. uncooked boneless, skinless chicken breasts
- 4 tablespoons light butter
- ½ cup chopped onion
- ¼ cup flour
- ½ teaspoon salt
- ¼ teaspoon black pepper
- 1 ½ cups skim milk
- 2 ½ cups water*
- 1 tablespoon Better Than Bouillon Roasted Chicken Base
- ½ teaspoon poultry seasoning
- 8 oz. uncooked egg noodles
- 1 cup frozen corn kernels
- 2 cups frozen peas and carrots

DIRECTIONS:

1. Place the chicken breasts in a Dutch oven or other large pot and cover with water to about 2 inches over the chicken.

2. Bring the water to a boil over high heat and then reduce the heat to medium. Cook over medium heat for 15-20 minutes (depending on the thickness of your chicken breasts – mine are generally done at 15, so check one then) until chicken is cooked through.

3. Remove the chicken breasts to a cutting board. Discard the water from the pot and rinse and wipe out the pot to use again. Chop the chicken into small, bite-size pieces and set aside.

4. Melt the butter in the pot over medium heat. Add the chopped onion and cook for a few minutes until the onion is softened.

5. Whisk in the flour, salt and pepper until combined with the butter and onions and continue to whisk for another 1-2 minutes.

6. Slowly whisk in the milk until combined and smooth. Add the water and bouillon base (or broth) and poultry seasoning and whisk in to combine.

7. Increase the heat to med-high and stir occasionally until boiling. Reduce the heat to med-low and add the egg noodles. Cook for 8 minutes, stirring regularly to prevent

sticking. If you need a little more liquid toward the end you can add a bit more water or broth.

8. Add the chopped chicken, corn, and peas and carrots and stir until thoroughly combined. Cook for another few minutes until all ingredients are heated through.

NUTRITION INFORMATION PER (1 ¼ CUP) SERVING:

314 calories, 35 g carbs, 3 g sugars, 7 g fat, 2 g saturated fat, 27 g protein, 3 g fiber

Yummy Whole Wheat Pasta and Spinach

Ready in 12 minutes.

8 servings,

Ingredients

- 1-pound whole wheat fusilli pasta

- 4 cups chopped spinach frozen

- 5 cups water

- 4 minced cloves garlic to taste

- Salt and pepper to taste

- 4 tablespoons butter, cut into cubes

- ½ cup Parmesan cheese, grated and more for serving

Instructions

1. Place pasta in Instant Pot bowl and 5 cups of water to cover. Add in garlic and frozen spinach. Select Manual (HIGH) setting and cook for 6 minutes.

2. Quick release pressure. Open the lid, stir and add salt, pepper, butter and Parmesan and cheese. Stir once more and put the lid back on and let pasta sit for 5 minutes.

3. Top with more Parmesan cheese.

Nutrition information

Calories: 293.4

Carbohydrates: 33.5g

Fats: 7.4g

Delicious Cheeseburger Soup

Cooking time: 2 hours

Serves: 4

Ingredients:

1 medium onion(chopped),

1 clove garlic(minced),

1 small stalk celery(chopped),

½ pound 93% lean ground beef,

½ cup low fat evaporated milk,

1 ½ cups chicken broth(divided),

4 ounces low fat Velveeta cheese(cubed),

Salt to taste,

Pepper to taste,

¼ teaspoon paprika to taste,

1 tablespoon all-purpose flour,

A dozen tortilla chips(crumbled)

and Cooking spray

INSTRUCTIONS:

1) Place a skillet over medium heat. Spray with cooking spray.

2) Add onion, garlic, and celery and sauté until translucent. Spray the inside of the slow cooker with cooking spray. Transfer the sautéed onions into it.

3) Place the skillet back on heat and add beef. Cook until the beef is brown. Break it simultaneously as it cooks. Transfer into the slow cooker.

4) Mix in bowl flour and a little broth and add it to the skillet.

5) Place the skillet back on heat. Insert the remaining broth and always stir until thick. Scrape any brown bits that were stuck to the bottom of the skillet.

6) Transfer into the slow cooker. Add cheese, salt, pepper and evaporated milk and stir.

7) Cover and set on 'Low' for 2 hours. Ladle into soup bowls. Top with tortilla chips and serve.

Scrumptious Delicious Grilled Salmon

COOKING TIME: 5 minutes

SERVES: 2

Ingredients:

¾ pound wild salmon fillet(skinless, chopped into 1 inch pieces),

½ teaspoon ground cumin,

Kosher salt to taste,

Olive oil cooking spray,

8 bamboo skewers soaked in water for an hour,

1 tablespoon fresh oregano(chopped),

¼ teaspoon red pepper flakes,

1 teaspoon sesame seeds,

1 lemon sliced into thin rounds

INSTRUCTIONS:

1) Preheat the grill to medium heat. Spray the grill grates with cooking spray. Mix together in a bowl, cumin, red pepper, sesame, and oregano and set aside.

2) Thread2 the salmon onto the skewers with the lemon slices in between.

3) Place the skewers on the grill and grill until the fish turns opaque.

Serve and enjoy.

Heavenly Pancakes

Ingredients:

1 tsp. sweetener, artificial

1 beaten egg white

½ Tbsp. cinnamon

½ Tbsp. baking powder

½ c. buttermilk

¾ c. whole wheat flour

1/3 c. unsweetened applesauce

Directions:

1. Combine together the egg, sweetener, cinnamon, baking powder, buttermilk, flour, and applesauce inside a bowl until there are no more lumps. Add in a bit of water to help the consistency if it is too thick.

2. Spray a bit of cooking spray on the skillet and let it heat up. When the skillet is ready, add a bit of the batter to the skillet and spread it out a bit.

3. Let these pancakes cook for a few minutes to allow the bubbles to start forming.

4. At this time, flip over the pancake and let it cook for an additional minute. Take off the heat when done and then repeat the steps with the rest of the batter until done.

Tasty Creamy-Tomato-Basil-Soup

Serves: 4

Ingredients

- 1 cup low sodium chicken broth
- 1 14 oz. can tomato puree
- 1 cup skim milk
- 4-5 leaves fresh basil
- 3 tsp. olive oil
- 1 stalk celery
- ½ cup onions
- 1 Tbsp. cornstarch
- 1-2 cloves garlic, crushed.
- pepper to taste

Instructions

1. Rough chop onions and celery, transfer them to a food processor or chopper and puree until fine.
2. Heat olive oil in a large pan over medium heat.
3. Add onion and celery mix to pan and sauté until they begin to become translucent.
4. Reduce heat to low and stir in garlic, pepper, chicken stock, and tomato puree, and cornstarch-simmer on low for 5 minutes.
5. Whisk in tomato puree and milk, top with basil leaves, simmer for an additional 10 minutes.
6. Serve topped with a dollop of Greek yogurt or a fresh chopped basil.
7. This makes approximately 4 -1/2 cup servings

Delicious Freestyle Chicken Parmesan

251 calories

TOTAL TIME: 30 minutes

Chicken Parmesan comes out great in the Air Fryer, no need to use so much oil!

INGREDIENTS:
- 2 (about 8 oz. each) chicken breast, fat trimmed, sliced in half to make 4
- 6 tbsp. seasoned breadcrumbs
- 2 tbsp. grated Parmesan cheese
- 1 tbsp. butter, melted (or olive oil)
- 6 tbsp. reduced fat mozzarella cheese
- 1/2 cup marinara
- cooking spray

DIRECTIONS:
1. Preheat the air fryer 360F° for 9 minutes. Spray the basked lightly with spray.
2. Combine breadcrumbs and parmesan cheese in a bowl. Melt the butter in another bowl.

3. Lightly brush the butter onto the chicken, then dip into breadcrumb mixture.
4. When the air fryer is ready, place 2 pieces in the basket and spray the top with oil.
5. Cook 6 minutes, turn and top each with 1 tbsp. sauce and 1 1/2 tbsp. of shredded mozzarella cheese.
6. Cook 3 more minutes or until cheese is melted.
7. Set aside and keep warm, repeat with the remaining 2 pieces.

NUTRITION INFORMATION

Yield: 4 servings,

Serving Size: 1 piece

Amount Per Serving:

- Calories: 251
- Total Fat: 9.5g
- Saturated Fat: g
- Sodium: mg
- Carbohydrates: 14g
- Fiber: 1.5g
- Sugar: 0g
- Protein: 31.5g

Yummy Baked potatoes in the instant pot

Ready in 30 minutes,

15 servings

Ingredients

- Potatoes, peeled or chopped (amount depends on personal preference). They should all be roughly of the same size.

Instructions

1. Add 1 cup of water into the pot and add in the potatoes

2. Tightly lid the pot and turn the sealing vent is turned to "sealed".

3. Cook for the next 10 minutes and let the pressure valve release naturally for 20 minutes.

4. Remove the lid and serve the potatoes.

Nutrition information

Calories: 161

Carbohydrates: 37g

Fats: 0.2g

Proteins: 4.3g

Delicious Vanilla Yogurt Scones

COOKING TIME: 5 minutes

SERVES: 3

INGREDIENTS:

2/3 cups of all-purpose flour,

1/3 cup of vanilla yogurt,

1 teaspoon of salt,

3 tablespoons of chopped peaches,

Non-stick cooking spray,

½ teaspoon of baking powder,

2 tablespoons of sugar,

1 teaspoon of margarine,

½ teaspoon of baking soda

and 1 teaspoon of powdered sugar

INSTRUCTIONS:

1) Preheat the oven to 400 degrees F

2) Take a medium size mixing bowl and add the flour, sugar (not powdered), baking powder, baking soda, and salt. Mix the ingredients and add in the margarine while doing so.

3) The margarine can be difficult to work with so you may want to heat it up in a microwave for 15 seconds.

4) Meanwhile, add the yogurt and the peaches, mixing while you do so.

5) Take a large piece of wax paper and empty the contents of the bowl onto the paper. Knead the dough for 4 minutes.

6) Coat a large baking tray with non-stick spray and form the scones on the tray. The scones look best when shaped like triangles.

7) The exact size of the scones is not as important as making sure the scones are of equal size. This recipe usually yields between 4 and 6 scones.

8) Make sure the dough is firmly pressed against the baking tray. Bake for 12-15 minutes on the center oven rack.

9) Remove the scones from the oven and while still hot, paint the scones with milk. This should look like they are slightly moist from the milk. Use this moisture to spread the powdered sugar over the scones.

Once done, serve and enjoy.

Scrumptious Freestyle Turkey Meatball & Veggie

Makes 8 servings.

One serving is 1-1/2 cups soup.

INGREDIENTS

- Cooking spray
- 1 onion, chopped
- 3-4 carrots, sliced or chopped
- 1 cup green beans, cut
- 2 minced garlic cloves
- 1 (24 ounce) package Jennie-O Italian style turkey meatballs
- 2 (14.5 ounce) cans beef or vegetable broth
- 2 (14.5 ounce) diced or Italian stewed tomatoes
- 1-1/2 cups frozen corn
- 1 teaspoon oregano
- 1 teaspoon parsley
- ½ teaspoon basil

INSTRUCTIONS

1. Spray large saucepan or instant pot with cooking spray.
2. Add onions, carrots, green beans and garlic and cook over medium heat 2-3 minutes.

3. Mix in remaining ingredients.

4. If cooking on a stovetop, cover and cook over medium-low heat for 20 minutes, or until meatballs are heated through.

5. -OR-

6. If using an instant pot, press the "soup" button and cook on high pressure for 15 minutes. Vent to release pressure once cooked.

7. -OR-

8. Cook in a slow cooker for 5-6 hours on LOW.

9. Serve warm.

10.   Refrigerate or freeze leftovers.

Nutrition Information

- Serves: 8 servings
- Serving size: 1-1/2 cup soup
- Calories: 285
- Fat: 13 g
- Saturated fat: 4 g
- Trans fat: 0 g
- Carbohydrates: 21 g
- Sugar: 9 g
- Sodium: 1126 mg
- Fiber: 3 g
- Protein: 19 g

Tasty Pizza Lasagna Roll-Ups

Yield: 8 PIECES

INGREDIENTS:

- 8 uncooked lasagna noodles
- 15 oz. can tomato sauce
- 1 cup pizza sauce
- ½ teaspoon Italian seasoning
- 1 lb. uncooked hot Italian poultry sausage, casings removed if present (I used Wegmans patties, you can use chicken or turkey sausage)
- 2 oz. turkey pepperoni, chopped (reserve 8 slices un-chopped for topping)
- 1 (15 oz.) container fat free Ricotta cheese
- 1 (10 oz.) package frozen chopped spinach, thawed and squeezed until dry
- 1 large egg
- 2 oz. 2% shredded Mozzarella cheese

INSTRUCTIONS:

Pre-heat the oven to 350. Lightly mist a 9×13 baking dish with cooking spray and set aside.

1. Boil and salt a large pot of water and cook lasagna noodles according to package instructions. Drain and rinse with cold water. Lay noodles flat on a clean dry surface and set aside.

2. In a mixing bowl, combine the tomato sauce, pizza sauce and Italian seasoning and stir together. Set aside.

3. Place the sausage in a large skillet over medium heat and cook until browned, breaking the meat up into small pieces as it cooks. When the sausage is cooked through, add the chopped pepperoni and 1/3 cup of the tomato sauce mixture and stir to combine. Remove from heat.

4. In a mixing bowl, combine the ricotta cheese, spinach and egg and stir until well combined. Spoon 1/3 cup of the cheese mixture onto each lasagna noodle and spread across the surface leaving a little room (about ½") at the far end with no toppings. Top the cheese layer on each noodle with the meat mixture from step four, evenly dividing the meat between the noodles. Starting with one end (not the one with space at the end), roll the noodle over the filling until it becomes a complete roll. Repeat with all noodles.

5. Spoon ½ cup of the tomato sauce mixture into the prepared baking dish and spread across the bottom. Place the lasagna rolls seam down in the dish and spoon or pour the remaining sauce over top. Sprinkle the Mozzarella over the top of the rolls and place a pepperoni on each one. Cover the dish with aluminum foil and bake for 40 minutes.

NUTRITION INFORMATION:

289 calories, 31 g carbs, 9 g sugars, 8 g fat, 2 g saturated fat, 24 g protein, 4 g fiber

Lunch

Tasty Freestyle Instant Pot Garlicky Cuban Pork

213 calories

TOTAL TIME: 80 minutes plus marinade time

Tender shredded pork, marinated in garlic, cumin, grapefruit and lime and cooked in the pressure cooker is perfect to serve over a bed of rice, cauliflower rice or with tortillas and salsa and avocados for taco night.

INGREDIENTS:

- 3 lb. boneless pork shoulder blade roast, lean, all fat removed
- 6 cloves garlic
- juice of 1 grapefruit (about 2/3 cup)
- juice of 1 lime
- 1/2 tablespoon fresh oregano
- 1/2 tablespoon cumin
- 1 tablespoon kosher salt
- 1 bay leaf
- lime wedges, for serving
- chopped cilantro, for serving
- hot sauce, for serving
- tortillas, optional for serving

- salsa, optional for serving

DIRECTIONS:
1. PRESSURE COOKER: Cut the pork in 4 pieces and place in a bowl.
2. In a small blender or mini food processor, combine garlic, grapefruit juice, lime juice, oregano, cumin and salt and blend until smooth.
3. Pour the marinade over the pork and let it sit room temperature 1 hour or refrigerated as long as overnight.
4. Transfer to the pressure cooker, add the bay leaf, cover and cook high pressure 80 minutes. Let the pressure release naturally.
5. Remove pork and shred using two forks.
6. Remove liquid from pressure cooker, reserving then place the pork back into pressure cooker. Add about 1 cup of the liquid (jus) back, adjust the salt as needed and keep warm until you're ready to eat.

SLOW COOKER:
1. Cut the pork in 4 pieces and place in a bowl.
2. In a small blender or mini food processor, combine garlic, grapefruit juice, lime juice, oregano, cumin and salt and blend until smooth.

3. Pour the marinade over the pork and let it sit room temperature 1 hour or refrigerated as long as overnight.

4. Transfer to the slow cooker, add the bay leaf, cover and cook low 8 hours.

5. Remove pork and shred using two forks.

6. Remove liquid from slow cooker, reserving then place the pork back into slow cooker. Add about 1 cup of the liquid (jus) back, adjust the salt as needed and keep warm until you're ready to eat.

NUTRITION INFORMATION

Yield: 10 servings, Serving Size: a little over 3 oz.

- Amount Per Serving:
- Calories: 213
- Total Fat: 9.5g
- Saturated Fat: 0g
- Sodium: 440.5mg
- Carbohydrates: 2.5g
- Fiber: 0.5g
- Sugar: 1.5g
- Protein: 26.5g

Delicious Pressure Cooker Texas Red Chili

Ready in 1 hour

6 servings

Ingredients

- 1 tablespoon vegetable oil
- 4-5 pounds' beef chuck roast, chopped 2 inch cubes
- ½ tablespoon kosher salt
- 2 onions, diced
- 3 cloves garlic, minced
- 2 minced chipotles with sauce
- 1/2 teaspoon kosher salt
- 1 teaspoon chili powder
- ½ cup cumin
- 2 teaspoons Mexican oregano
- 1 cup coffee
- 14 ounces can of crushed tomatoes
- Salt and pepper to taste

Instructions

1. Brown the beef: Heat the oil in the cooker pot over medium-high heat for 30 seconds. Sprinkle the beef with salt and then brown in two to three batches. Brown each batch on one side, about five minutes.

2. Add in the onions and 1/2 teaspoon of kosher salt to the cooker. Fry the onions for about 5 minutes until softened while scraping with a spoon to remove any stuck bits on the bottom. Add the garlic cloves and chipotle and then fry for one minute. Add the chili powder, oregano and cumin. Allow to cook for one minute and then stir the spices into the onions.

3. Pour the beef and any juices into the cooker, and then add the crushed tomatoes. Stir until the beef is completely coated in tomatoes and spices.

4. Shut the cooker tightly, bring the high heat and maximum pressure. Cook for 25 minutes and then release pressure naturally, about 15 minutes and then remove the lid.

5. Add salt to reduce chili bitterness. Serve the chili straight up.

Nutrition information

Calories: 225

Carbohydrates: 7g

Fats: 16g

Proteins: 14g

Heavenly Chicken and Pancetta Risotto and black pepper and lemon

Ready in 18-20 minutes,

4 servings

Ingredients:

- 1 large onion, chopped
- 2 garlic cloves, chopped
- 100g butter
- 1 tablespoon olive oil
- ½ tablespoon salt
- ½ tablespoon black pepper
- ½ tablespoon pancetta, diced
- 300g diced chicken
- 1 cup Arborio rice
- 4 tablespoon grated parmesan
- ½ cup white wine
- 2 cups chicken stock
- 1 tablespoon fresh thyme
- ½ tablespoon parmesan grated
- Black pepper, freshly ground

- 1 lemon grated zest
- Basil leaves

Directions:
1. Select 'fry' setting to preheat Instant Pot, and add the oil, and 30g of butter to the pan. Fry onions, garlic, pancetta and chicken for 2 minutes.
2. Stir in rice and season well, add thyme, and stir in the wine. Stop the pot. Pour in the stock and stir well.
3. Press the 'Manual' cooking button and adjust the cooking time to 12 minutes. Stir the risotto one last time and seal the pot with lid.
4. When the cooking time is over, stir the risotto to develop the creamy texture, and stir in the grated parmesan, and the remaining butter. Allow to for 3 minutes.
5. Top with extra parmesan, freshly ground black pepper basil leaves and grated lemon zest and serve.

Nutrition information
Calories: 582.7
Carbohydrates: 77.3g

Fats: 13.4g

Proteins: 35.1g

Irresistible Freestyle Buffalo Wing Hummus

Yield: 8 (1/4 CUP) SERVINGS

INGREDIENTS:

- 1 ½ cups canned chickpeas, drained and rinsed (reserve ¼ cup of the liquid from the can)
- 2 cloves garlic
- 2 tablespoons tahini
- 2 tablespoons fresh lemon juice
- ¾ teaspoon paprika
- 1 tablespoon barbecue sauce
- 1 ½ tablespoons Frank's Red Hot (or similar cayenne pepper sauce)
- 1 ½ teaspoons white vinegar
- ¾ teaspoon salt

DIRECTIONS:

1. Combine all ingredients including the ¼ reserved liquid from the can of chickpeas into a food processor or blender. Puree ingredients until smooth. Serve.

NUTRITION INFORMATION:

72 calories, 12 g carbs, 1 g sugars, 2 g fat, 0 g saturated fat, 3 g protein, 2 g fiber

Mouthwatering Leftover Turkey and Sweet Potato Frittata

COOKING TIME: 25 minutes

SERVES: 3

INGREDIENTS:

2 large egg whites,

3 large eggs,

½ ounce Gruyere cheese(grated),

6 ounces sweet potatoes(chopped into ½ inch pieces),

1 small onion(chopped),

½ cup baby spinach(chopped),

3 ounces leftover turkey breast(cut),

Freshly ground black pepper,

½ teaspoon kosher salt or to taste,

1 teaspoon olive oil,

¼ teaspoon dried thyme,

¼ teaspoon paprika,

and 1/8 teaspoon garlic powder

INSTRUCTIONS:

1) Whisk together eggs, whites, 1/8-teaspoon salt, and pepper. Add cheese and stir.

2) Place an ovenproof skillet over medium heat. Add oil. When the oil is heated, add onions and sauté until golden. Add sweet potatoes, thyme, garlic powder, paprika, some more salt, and pepper and stir. Cover and cook until tender and crisp as well.

3) Add turkey and stir. Add spinach and cook until it wilts.

4) Lower heat. Pour the eggs into it. Cook for 6-7 minutes until the edges begin to set.

5) Transfer the skillet to a preheated oven. Bake in a preheated oven at 400° F for about 10 minutes or a toothpick, when inserted in the center, comes out clean. Let it remain in the oven for about 10 minutes.

Slice into wedges and serve.

Yummy Mediterranean Bean Salad

COOKING TIME: 30 minutes

SERVES: 3

INGREDIENTS:

7.5 ounces canned black beans(drained, rinsed),

7.5 ounces canned garbanzo beans(drained, rinsed),

1 clove garlic(minced),

2 tablespoons fresh mint(chopped),

2 tablespoons fresh parsley(chopped),

½ cup grape tomatoes(chopped),

¼ cup red onion(chopped),

Juice of ½ lemon,

2 teaspoons olive oil,

Freshly ground pepper to taste and Kosher salt to taste

INSTRUCTIONS:

1) Add olive oil and lemon juice to a small bowl and whisk until emulsified. Add all the remaining ingredients of the salad into a bowl and mix.

2) Pour dressing over it. Toss well and set aside for 30 minutes at room temperature.

Toss well and serve

Mouth Watering Freestyle Sticky Buffalo Chicken Tenders

Prep time: 10 mins

Cook time: 15 mins

Total time: 25 mins

Ingredients

- 1 pound boneless skinless chicken breasts, pounded to ½" thickness
- ¼ cup flour
- 3 eggs
- 1 cup Italian Seasoned Panko breadcrumbs
- ½ cup brown sugar
- ⅓ cup Frank's Red Hot Sauce
- ½ teaspoon Garlic Powder
- 3 tablespoons water

INSTRUCTIONS:

1. Preheat oven to 425 degrees and spray a baking sheet with non-stick cooking spray or line with silicone baking mats.

2. Cut boneless skinless chicken breasts into strips or chunks (we find chunks hold coating better).

3. Add the chicken into a large Ziploc bag that contains just the flour. Shake to coat.

4. Place Panko breadcrumbs into a shallow bowl. In another shallow bowl, whisk eggs until combined well.

5. Dip flour coated chicken into eggs, then into Panko breadcrumbs to coat.

6. Place coated chicken on the prepared baking sheet. Spray tops with non-stick cooking spray.

7. Bake for 15 minutes for nuggets or 20 minutes for strips or until chicken is browned and cooked through.

8. While chicken is in the oven, you will make your sauce mixture.

9. In a medium saucepan, bring the brown sugar, garlic powder, water and Frank's red hot sauce to a boil. Remove from heat and stir well.

10. When chicken is cooked through, remove from the oven and toss with sauce. This will just coat the chicken.

Heavenly Apple Muffin

Ingredients:

½ c. milk

2 Tbsp. vegetable oil

½ tsp. salt

½ tsp. cinnamon

1 ½ tsp. baking powder

1 c. oats

½ tsp. baking soda

2/3 c. brown sugar

2 c. shredded apple

1 ½ c. flour, all purpose

Directions:

1. Turn on the oven and let it heat up to 375 degrees. In the meantime, take out a muffin pan and grease it up.

2. Take out a bowl and combine together the milk, cinnamon, vegetable oil, baking soda, salt, brown sugar, baking powder, flour, and oats.

3. When this is all combined, pour the batter inside the muffin tin and then place into the oven.

4. Allow these to bake for 18 minutes or until they are all done. Give them some time to cool down before serving.

Delicious Watering Instant pot Mexican beef

Ready in 50 minutes,

6 servings

Ingredients

- 3 pounds' boneless beef short ribs sliced into cubes
- ½ cup chili powder
- 2 teaspoons salt
- 1 tablespoon fat
- 1 medium onion, thinly sliced
- 2 tablespoon tomato paste
- 5 garlic cloves, well peeled and smashed
- ½ cup roasted tomato salsa
- ½-1 cup bone broth
- 1 teaspoon Red Boat Fish Sauce
- black pepper, freshly ground
- ½ cup minced cilantro
- 2 radishes, thinly sliced

Instructions

1. Combine the cubed beef, chili powder, and salt in a large bowl.

2. Bring pot to medium heat and when the fat melts, add the onions then sauté until soft.

3. Stir in tomato paste and garlic, and cook until fragrant or 30 seconds.

4. Add in the seasoned beef then pour in the salsa, fish sauce and stock.

5. Tight lid the pot and cook on high heat until high pressure is reached. Afterwards, lower the heat to maintain high pressure for about 30 minutes. Release pressure naturally for 15 minutes.

6. Unlock the lid, season with salt and pepper to taste and serve.

Nutrition information

Calories: 209.5

Carbohydrates: 6.8g

Fats: 13.4g

Proteins: 15.1g

Scrumptious Pork chops and cabbage

Ready in 20 minutes

4 servings

Ingredients

- 4 pork chops, thick cut
- 1-2 teaspoon of fennel seeds
- ½ tablespoon salt
- 1 teaspoon pepper
- 1 small head of cabbage
- ¾ cup meat stock
- 1 tablespoon vegetable oil
- 2 teaspoons flour

Instructions

1. Sprinkle the pork chops with fennel, pepper and salt.
2. Slicing the cabbage into half, and then into thick ¾ inch slices then set aside.

3. Heat oil to the pre-heated pressure cooker over medium-high heat and brown all the chops and then set aside. Afterwards, add in the cabbage slices to the empty pressure cooker.

4. Arrange the pork chops on top of the cabbage brown-side up. Add in any juice from the chops.

5. Cover the cooker with lid and bring pressure to high heat and pressure. Turn up the heat high and then lower to maintain pressure. Cook for the next 6-8 minutes at high pressure.

6. Afterwards, open the cooker gently by slowly releasing the pressure.

7. Extract the cabbage and pork chops onto a serving platter. Bring the remaining juices in the pressure cooker to boil and then whisk-in the flour.

8. Pour the thickened sauce on the cabbage and pork chops platter and then serve.

Nutrition information

Calories: 366

Carbohydrates: 22g

Fats: 22g

Proteins: 20g

Tasty Freestyle Sticky Buffalo Chicken Tenders

Prep time: 10 mins

Cook time: 15 mins

Total time: 25 mins

Ingredients

- 1 pound boneless skinless chicken breasts, pounded to ½" thickness
- ¼ cup flour
- 3 eggs
- 1 cup Italian Seasoned Panko breadcrumbs
- ½ cup brown sugar
- ⅓ cup Frank's Red Hot Sauce
- ½ teaspoon Garlic Powder
- 3 tablespoons water

Instructions

1. Preheat oven to 425 degrees and spray a baking sheet with non-stick cooking spray or line with silicone baking mats.

2. Cut boneless skinless chicken breasts into strips or chunks (we find chunks hold coating better).

3. Add the chicken into a large Ziploc bag that contains just the flour. Shake to coat.

4. Place Panko breadcrumbs into a shallow bowl. In another shallow bowl, whisk eggs until combined well.

5. Dip flour coated chicken into eggs, then into Panko breadcrumbs to coat.

6. Place coated chicken on the prepared baking sheet. Spray tops with non-stick cooking spray.

7. Bake for 15 minutes for nuggets or 20 minutes for strips or until chicken is browned and cooked through.

8. While chicken is in the oven, you will make your sauce mixture.

9. In a medium saucepan, bring the brown sugar, garlic powder, water and Frank's red hot sauce to a boil. Remove from heat and stir well.

10. When chicken is cooked through, remove from the oven and toss with sauce. This will just coat the chicken.

Irresistible Freestyle White Chicken Chili

Yield: 8 (1 CUP) SERVINGS

INGREDIENTS:

- 1 tablespoon Canola oil
- 2 cups yellow onion, chopped
- 2 tablespoons chili powder
- 1 tablespoon minced garlic
- 2 teaspoons ground cumin
- 1 teaspoon oregano
- 3 (15.5 oz.) cans Great Northern beans, rinsed and drained
- 4 cups reduced sodium fat free chicken broth
- 3 cups chopped or shredded cooked skinless chicken breast
- 1 (14.5 oz.) can diced tomatoes

- 1/3 cup chopped fresh cilantro
- 2 tablespoon fresh lime juice
- ½ teaspoon salt
- ½ teaspoon pepper

DIRECTIONS:

1. Bring oil to medium heat in a large pot or Dutch oven. Add the onions and sauté for 5-8 minutes or until tender.

2. Add the chili powder, garlic and cumin and stir to coat the onions. Cook for 2 more minutes. Add the oregano and beans, stir and cook for 30 more seconds.

3. Add the broth and reduce the heat to medium-low. Simmer for 20 minutes, stirring occasionally.

4. Remove 2 cups of the bean/broth mixture into a blender (or container for an immersion blender) and process until smooth.

5. Return pureed mixture to the pot. Add the chicken and tomatoes and cook over medium-low for another 30 minutes, stirring occasionally.

6. Add the cilantro, lime juice, salt & pepper and stir to combine before serving.

NUTRITION INFORMATION PER 1 CUP SERVING:
291 calories, 36 g carbs, 4 g sugars, 4 g fat, 1 g saturated fat, 27 g protein, 12 g fiber

Scrumptious Freestyle Chicken MeatBall

248 calories

TOTAL TIME: 30 minutes

INGREDIENTS:

- 8 ounces sliced cremini mushrooms, divided
- 1 pound 93% lean ground chicken
- 1/3 cup whole wheat seasoned or gluten-free bread crumbs
- 1/4 cup grated Pecorino cheese
- 1 large egg, beaten
- 3 garlic cloves, minced
- 2 tablespoons chopped fresh parsley, plus more for garnish
- 1 teaspoon Kosher salt
- Freshly ground black pepper
- 1/2 tablespoon all-purpose flour
- 1/2 tablespoon unsalted butter
- 1/4 cup finely chopped shallots
- 3 ounces sliced shiitake mushrooms
- 1/3 cup Marsala wine
- 3/4 cup reduced sodium chicken broth

DIRECTIONS:

1. Preheat the oven to 400F.
2. Finely chop half of the Cremini mushrooms and transfer to a medium bowl with the ground chicken, breadcrumbs, Pecorino, egg, 1 clove of the minced garlic, parsley, 1 teaspoon kosher salt and black pepper, to taste.
3. Gently shape into 25 small meatballs, bake 15 to 18 minutes, until golden.
4. In a small bowl whisk the flour with the Marsala wine and broth.
5. Heat a large skillet on medium heat.
6. Add the butter, garlic and shallots and cook until soft and golden, about 2 minutes.
7. Add the mushrooms, season with 1/8 teaspoon salt and a pinch of black pepper, and cook, stirring occasionally, until golden, about 5 minutes.
8. Return the meatballs to the pot, pour the Marsala wine mixture over the meatballs, cover and cook 10 minutes.
9. Garnish with parsley.

NUTRITION INFORMATION

Yield: 5 servings, Serving Size: 5 meatballs with mushrooms

Mouth Watering Watermelon, Jicama, & Cucumber Salad

COOKING TIME:

SERVES: 3

INGREDIENTS:

1 tablespoon olive oil,

Juice of ½ lime,

Freshly ground black pepper to taste,

Kosher salt to taste,

1 teaspoon raw honey,

1 cup jicama peeled(cubed),

1 cup watermelon(deseeded, cubed),

1 small red onion (thinly sliced),

1 medium cucumber(peeled, deseeded, cubed),

1 tablespoon fresh mint (chopped)

and 1-ounce feta cheese (crumbled or chopped into small cubes)

INSTRUCTIONS:

1) Add all the ingredients for the dressing in a small bowl and whisk until well combined.

2) Add all the salad ingredients into a bowl and toss. Pour the dressing over it and toss well.

Serve.

Scrumptious Scallion Cheesy Bell Pepper Bake

COOKING TIME: 30 minutes

SERVES: 4

INGREDIENTS:

2 large white eggs,

4 large eggs,

5 ounces frozen chopped spinach (thawed, squeezed of excess moisture),

1/3 cup canned artichokes (drained, pat dried),

¼ cup scallions (finely chopped),

1 clove garlic (minced),

3 tablespoons red bell pepper (chopped),

2 teaspoons fresh dill (chopped),

2 tablespoons fat-free milk, ¼ cup feta cheese (crumbled),

1 tablespoon parmesan cheese (grated), Salt to taste, Pepper to taste and Cooking spray

INSTRUCTIONS:

1) Spray a baking dish with cooking spray. Add spinach, scallions, artichoke, red pepper and garlic into it. Mix well and spread all over the dish evenly.

2) Whisk together in a bowl, eggs, whites, milk, salt, and pepper. Add Parmesan and feta and stir. Pour over the vegetables in the dish.

3) Bake in a preheated oven at 375° F for about 30 minutes or a toothpick, when inserted in the center, comes out clean.

Slice into wedges and serve.

Enjoy.

Delicious Mushroom and Spinach Quiche

Ingredients:

Salt

Pepper

¼ c. chopped onion

3 eggs

½ c. cottage cheese

2 tsp. garlic, minced

1 c. artichoke hearts, chopped

½ tsp. olive oil

10 oz. spinach

1 c. mushrooms, sliced

Directions:

1. Turn on the oven and let it heat up to 350 degrees. While that is heating up, take out a pan and cook together the olive oil, mushrooms, onions, and garlic.

2. When those are ready, add in the spinach and let it cook for a bit. After a few minutes, add in the rest of the ingredients and season with some pepper and salt.

3. Place this into a prepared pie dish and let it bake for 45 minutes before serving.

Heavenly Freestyle Scalloped, Ham & Potatoes

Prep Time

45 mins

Cook Time

7 hrs.

Total Time

7 hrs. 45 mins

Slow cooker scalloped potatoes and ham, a comforting classic dish made lighter your whole family will love.

Course: Main

Servings:

Calories: 249 kcal

Tasty Whole Chicken in an Instant Pot

Ready in 55 minutes,

6 servings

Ingredients

- 1 whole chicken
- Any preferred seasonings
- 1 cup water
- 1 tablespoon coconut oil

Directions

1. Put a cup of water into the Instant Pot and add in the steam rack.
2. Heat the oil in a large skillet.
3. Coat the chicken with seasonings and then place in the oil and allow to brown for at least one minute on each side and then withdraw from heat.
4. Transfer the chicken to the Instant Pot on the steam rack.
5. Tight lid the Instant Pot and set to Chicken on high pressure. Adjust the time. Allow chicken to cook for

not more than 30 minutes and the release steam naturally for 15 minutes.You can as well save the bones and make broth instead of throwing them.

Nutrition information

Calories: 339

Carbohydrates: 1g

Fats: 19g

Proteins: 38g

Heavenly Cooker Cassoulete

Ready in 40 minutes,

4 servings

Ingredients

- 2 tablespoons olive oil
- 2 pounds of boneless pork ribs, chopped into bite size pieces
- Salt and pepper
- 2 cups beans, great northern
- 1 cup of beef broth
- 1 carrot, diced
- 1 diced celery stalk
- ½ diced white onion
- 2 tablespoons, dried rosemary
- 4 minced cloves garlic
- 2 cups herbed croutons
- 1 cup crumbled goat cheese

Instructions:

1. Heat the olive oil in a skillet over medium high heat. Sprinkle the pork ribs with salt and pepper, and then brown on all sides in the skillet.

2. Add the pork into the Instant Pot Pressure Cooker, and then add the beans, broth, garlic, carrot, celery, onion and rosemary. Seal the cooker, select the stew setting and cook for 35 minutes.

3. Divide cassoulet into 4 large soup bowls, top with croutons and goat cheese and serve.

Nutrition information

Calories: 540

Carbohydrates: 54g

Fats: 18g

Proteins: 35g

Tasty Scalloped Potatoes & Ham

Ingredients

- 8 cups peeled and thinly sliced potatoes (8 to 10 medium)
- Salt and pepper to taste
- 1 medium onion, sliced thin (about 1 cup)
- 1-1/2 cups cubed cooked ham
- 1 cup grated low-fat cheddar cheese
- 1 can (10-1/2 ounces) low-fat cream of mushroom soup (I used Campbell's Healthy Request)
- Paprika

Instructions

1. Ideal slow cooker size: 4- to 5-Quart.
2. Grease your slow cooker with nonstick cooking spray.
3. Put half the sliced potatoes in the bottom of your slow cooker, spreading them out evenly. Sprinkle with salt and pepper to taste.
4. Sprinkle evenly with half the onion, ham and cheese.
5. Repeat the layers one more time (potatoes, salt and pepper, onion, ham, cheese).
6. Pour the soup into a small bowl and stir it until it gets nice and creamy. Spread it over the top of the ingredients in the slow cooker.
7. Cover and cook on LOW for 6 to 8 hours, or until the potatoes and onions are tender when pierced with a fork.

8. Just before serving, sprinkle with a little paprika.

Nutrition Facts

Amount per Serving (1 cup)

Calories 249Calories from Fat 30

% Daily Value*

Total Fat 3.3g**5%**

Total Carbohydrates 40.4g**13%**

Dietary Fiber 5.7g**23%**

Protein 14.3g**29%**

* Percent Daily Values are based on a 2000 calorie diet.

Irresistible Burrito Bowl with Spiced Butternut Squash

COOKING TIME: 25 minutes

SERVES: 2

INGREDIENTS:

10 ounces butternut squash(deseeded, chopped into 1-inch cubes),

2 large eggs,

1 small onion(chopped),

½ cup tomatoes(chopped),

2 ounces Hass avocado(cubed),

1 teaspoon olive oil,

¼ teaspoon smoked paprika,

1 ½ teaspoons garlic powder,

Freshly ground pepper to taste,

Salt to taste,

14 teaspoon ground cumin,

1 teaspoon lime juice,

2 tablespoons fresh cilantro(chopped),

2 tablespoons low-fat cheddar cheese(shredded)

and Cooking spray

INSTRUCTIONS:

1) Grease a nonstick baking sheet with cooking spray. Add squash, oil, garlic powder, cumin, paprika, salt and pepper into a bowl. Toss well. Transfer onto the prepared baking sheet.

2) Bake in a preheated oven at 425° F for about 20-25 minutes until tender. Toss once halfway through baking.

3) Meanwhile, mix in a bowl, onions, tomatoes, cilantro, lime juice, salt, and pepper. Set aside for a while. Place a skillet over medium heat. Spray with cooking spray. Add eggs, sprinkle salt and pepper. Cook according to the way you like the eggs set.

4) To assemble: Divide and place squash in 2 bowls. Layer with the onion mixture followed by avocado slices. Next, put the egg over it. Sprinkle cheese over it and serve.

Delicious Spicy Lemon Chicken

COOKING TIME: 8 minutes

SERVES: 1

INGREDIENTS:

1 tbsp olive oil,

1/2 tsp red chili powder,

1/4 cup fresh lime juice,

3 chicken breast (boneless and skinless),

1 cup spicy salsa,

1/2 cup feta cheese (crumbled)

and 1/2 tsp ground cumin

INSTRUCTIONS:

1) Add olive oil in instant pot and select sauté.

2) Place chicken breasts in a pot for lightly brown both the sides.

3) Transfer chicken to a plate.

4) Then add cumin, chili powder, salsa and lime juice to the pot. Stir well and return the chicken to the pot.

5) Sealed pot with lid and Select manual high pressure for 8 minutes. After 8 minutes open pot lid using quick release method.

6) Transfer chicken breast and its sauce to a plate and sprinkle crumbled cheese and serve.

Enjoy.

Yummy Freestyle Slow Cook Chicken Cacciatore

INGREDIENTS:

- 8 bone-in, skinless chicken thighs
- 3/4 teaspoon kosher salt
- freshly ground black pepper
- cooking spray
- 5 garlic cloves, finely chopped
- 1/2 large onion, chopped
- 1 28-ounce can crushed tomatoes
- 1/2 medium red bell pepper, chopped
- 1/2 medium green bell pepper, chopped
- 4 ounce sliced shiitake mushrooms
- 1 sprig of fresh thyme
- 1 sprig of fresh oregano
- 1 bay leaf
- 1 tablespoon chopped fresh parsley (I omitted this)
- freshly grated Parmesan cheese, for serving (optional)

DIRECTIONS:

1. Season the chicken with salt and pepper to taste. Heat a large nonstick skillet over medium-high heat.
2. Coat with cooking spray, add the chicken, and cook until browned- 2 to 3 minutes per side. Transfer to your slow cooker.
3. Reduce the heat under the skillet to medium and coat with more cooking spray. Add the garlic and onion and cook, stirring, until soft- 3 to 4 minutes.
4. Transfer to the slow cooker and add the tomatoes, bell peppers, mushrooms, thyme, oregano and bay leaf. Stir to combine.
5. Cover and cook on high for 4 hours or on low for 8 hours.
6. Discard the bay leaf and transfer the chicken to a large plate. Pull the chicken meat from the bones (discard the bones), shred the meat, and return it to the sauce.
7. Stir in the parsley (if using). If desired, serve topped with Parmesan cheese.

Nutritional information per serving:

Calories: 220,

Fat: 6g,

Sat Fat: 1.5g,

Cholesterol: 123mg,

Sodium: 319mg,

Carbohydrates: 10g,

Fiber: 2g,

Sugar: 6g,

Protein: 31g

Delicious Freestyle Bruschetta Topped Balsamic Chicken

Yield: 4 SERVINGS

INGREDIENTS:

- 4 (6 oz.) raw boneless skinless chicken breasts or cutlets
- Salt and pepper, to taste
- ½ teaspoon dried oregano
- 2 teaspoons olive oil, divided
- ¾ cup balsamic vinegar
- 2 tablespoons sugar
- ¼ teaspoon salt
- 1 cup chopped cherry or grape tomatoes
- 1-2 tablespoons of sliced fresh basil
- 1 teaspoon minced garlic (or more to taste)

INSTRUCTIONS:

1. Pre-heat the oven to 400 degrees. Place the chicken breasts on a cutting board and if necessary, pound with a meat mallet to ensure an even thickness.

2. Sprinkle each breast with salt, pepper and oregano on each side.

3. Pour 1 ½ teaspoons of olive oil into a large skillet and bring over medium-high heat.

4. Place the breasts in the pan in a single layer and cook for 1-2 minutes on each side to lightly brown the outside of the chicken.

5. Mist a baking sheet with cooking spray and place the chicken breasts onto the sheet. Cover with aluminum foil and bake for 15 minutes.

6. While the chicken is baking, combine the balsamic vinegar, sugar and salt in a small saucepan and stir to combine. Bring to a boil over medium-high heat and then reduce the heat to medium low. Simmer for 10-15 minutes until the mixture has reduced and thickened and will coat the back of a spoon. Split the balsamic glaze into two small dishes.

7. When the chicken comes out of the oven, discard any extra liquid produced by the chicken. Use a pastry brush to brush the glaze from one of the dishes onto the chicken breasts. Place the baking sheet of chicken back in the oven, uncovered this time, for 5-10 minutes until the chicken is cooked through. Wash your pastry brush thoroughly.
8. Combine the chopped tomatoes, sliced basil, minced garlic and the remaining ½ teaspoon of olive oil in a bowl and add salt and pepper to taste. Stir to combine.
9. When the chicken breasts are done cooking, brush the second dish of balsamic glaze over the chicken breasts. Serve each breast topped with ¼ cup of the bruschetta tomato mixture.

NUTRITION INFORMATION:

293 calories, 18 g carbs, 17 g sugars, 7 g fat, 1 g saturated fat, 39 g protein, 1 g fiber .

Yummy Maple Smoked Brisket

Ready in 1 hr. 30 minutes

8 servings

Ingredients

- 1 lb. beef brisket
- 1-2 tablespoons maple, date, or coconut sugar,
- 2 teaspoons sea salt, smoked
- 1 teaspoon black pepper
- 1 teaspoon mustard powder
- 1 teaspoon onion powder
- ½ teaspoon smoked paprika
- 2 cups bone broth
- 3 fresh thyme sprigs

Instructions

1. Withdraw the brisket from refrigerator 30 minutes before cooking. Dry it with paper towels and set aside.

2. Combine the maple sugar, pepper, smoked sea salt, onion powder, mustard powder, and smoked paprika. Coat the meat with the mixture on all sides.

3. Add to the Instant Pot and allow it to fry for 2-3 minutes until golden brown. Turn the brisket and add the broth, thyme and liquid smoke. Scrape any browned bits at the bottom and then cover with the lid.

4. Allow to cook for 50 minutes and release steam naturally. Withdraw the brisket from the pot cover with foil and set aside. Slice the brisket and serve it.

Nutrition information

Calories: 542.9

Carbohydrates: 30.3g

Fats: 24g

Proteins: 45.6g

Tasty Freestyle Garlic Roasted Garbanzo Beans

Prep time: 5 mins

Cook time: 45 mins

Total time: 50 mins

Ingredients

- 1 can garbanzo beans (chickpeas)
- 1 tablespoon olive oil
- 1 teaspoon salt
- 1 teaspoon garlic powder
- ½ teaspoon paprika

Instructions

1. Preheat oven to 375° Fahrenheit.
2. Line a baking sheet with a silicone baking mat or parchment paper.
3. Drain and rinse the garbanzo beans.
4. Pat garbanzo beans dry, pour into a large bowl.
5. Toss with olive oil, salt, garlic powder, and paprika until all are well coated.
6. Spread evenly over baking sheet.
7. Bake at 375° for 20 minutes. Turn chickpeas so they are evenly roasted (use a spatula to flip them or simply stir around but make sure they are in an even layer).
8. Place back in the oven at 375° for additional 25 minutes.

9. Allow the roasted garbanzo beans to cool before storing in an airtight container for snacking.

Dinner

Yummy Freestyle Roasted Sweet Potato Side Dish

Prep time: 5 mins

Cook time: 25 mins

Total time: 30 mins

Ingredients

- 2 Medium Sweet Potatoes
- ½ teaspoon salt
- Non-Stick Cooking Spray

Instructions

1. Preheat oven to 400 degrees.
2. Line baking sheet with silicone baking mat or spray with non-stick spray.
3. Clean sweet potatoes, and peel if desired. We usually leave the skin intact. Remove any blemishes or eyes if needed.
4. Slice sweet potatoes into ¼" thick medallions
5. Place sweet potatoes in a single layer on prepared baking sheet.
6. Sprinkle the tops lightly with salt.
7. Bake at 400 degrees for 15 minutes. Turn sweet potato medallions over and bake additional 10 minutes.

Delicious Pressure Cooker Red Beans and Rice

Ready in 8 hrs. 45 minutes,

8 servings

Ingredients

- Beans and soaking
- Pound beans, well sorted and rinsed
- 1 tablespoon kosher salt
- 2 quarts' water
- Aromatics
- 2 teaspoon vegetable oil
- 1 pound smoked sausage quartered into 1/4 inch wedges
- 1 large onion, minced
- 1 stalk celery, minced
- 1 green bell pepper, seeded and minced
- 4 cloves garlic, thinly sliced
- 1 teaspoon fresh thyme leaves
- 1 teaspoon salt
- 2 bay leaves
- 1 teaspoon salt
- 5 cups water

- salt and pepper

- For serving

- Cooked long grain white rice

- Parsley minced

- Green onions, minced

- Hot sauce

Directions

1. Sort the beans, and remove broken beans, dirt and stones. Rinse and transfer into a large container add one tablespoon of salt and cover with 2 quarts' water.

2. Heat oil in the pressure cooker over medium heat until it shimmers and add the smoked sausage, garlic, onion, celery, bell pepper, thyme and sprinkle with salt. fry for 8 minutes until the onions and sausage turn brown around the edges.

3. Drain the beans and rinse. Pour them into the pressure cooker, add bay leaves and 1 teaspoon of salt, and then stir in the water. Tightly lid the pressure cooker and allow to cook at high pressure for the next 15 minutes. Release pressure naturally for about 20 minutes. Carefully remove the lid.

4. Discard the bay leaves. Scoop out 2 cups of the beans and the liquid, puree, and pour back into the pot.

Simmer for another fifteen minutes. Taste to check seasoning and serve.

Nutrition information

Calories: 838, Carbohydrates: 140g, Fats: 20g, Proteins: 23g

Mouth Watering Freestyle Marinara Spinach manicotti

277 calories

COOK TIME: 25 minutes

INGREDIENTS:

- 16 homemade crespelles
- 15 oz. part skim ricotta cheese (I use Polly-O)
- 2 cups shredded part-skim mozzarella cheese (reserve 1/2 cup) Polly-O
- 1 large egg
- 10 oz. package frozen spinach, thawed and squeezed really well
- 1/4 cup grated Parmesan Regianno
- 1/2 teaspoon kosher salt
- black pepper, to taste
- 2 1/2 cups jarred marinara
  DIRECTIONS:

1. Start by making the crespelles
2. Preheat oven to 375°F.
3. In a large bowl, combine ricotta, 1-1/2 cups of the mozzarella, egg, spinach, parmesan cheese, 1/2 teaspoon salt and pepper.
4. Fill each crespelle with 1/4 cup spinach filling and roll.

5. In a large baking dish, (or two smaller dishes) pour 1 cup of sauce on the bottom of the dish.

6. Place rolled manicotti seem side down onto baking dish. Top with 1 1/2 cups more sauce and remaining mozzarella cheese.

7. Cover with foil and bake about about 25 minutes, until hot and bubbling, and the cheese is melted.

NUTRITION INFORMATION

Yield: 8 servings, Serving Size: 2 manicotti

- Amount Per Serving:
- Calories: 277
- Total Fat: 12.5g
- Saturated Fat: 6g
- Sodium: 698mg
- Carbohydrates: 20g
- Fiber: 3g
- Sugar: 5g
- Protein: 22.5g

Tasty Turkey Meatball & Veggie Soup

Nutrition Information

- Serves: 8 servings
- Serving size: 1-1/2 cup soup
- Calories: 285
- Fat: 13 g
- Saturated fat: 4 g
- Trans fat: 0 g
- Carbohydrates: 21 g
- Sugar: 9 g
- Sodium: 1126 mg
- Fiber: 3 g
- Protein: 19 g

Makes 8 servings.

One serving is 1-1/2 cups soup.

One serving is 5 FreeStyle WW SP.

INGREDIENTS

- Cooking spray
- 1 onion, chopped

- 3-4 carrots, sliced or chopped
- 1 cup green beans, cut
- 2 minced garlic cloves
- 1 (24 ounce) package Jennie-O Italian style turkey meatballs
- 2 (14.5 ounce) cans beef or vegetable broth
- 2 (14.5 ounce) diced or Italian stewed tomatoes
- 1-1/2 cups frozen corn
- 1 teaspoon oregano
- 1 teaspoon parsley
- ½ teaspoon basil

INSTRUCTIONS

1. Spray large saucepan or instant pot with cooking spray.
2. Add onions, carrots, green beans and garlic and cook over medium heat 2-3 minutes.
3. Mix in remaining ingredients.
4. If cooking on a stovetop, cover and cook over medium-low heat for 20 minutes, or until meatballs are heated through.

   -OR-

5. If using an instant pot, press the "soup" button and cook on high pressure for 15 minutes. Vent to release pressure once cooked.

   -OR-

6. Cook in a slow cooker for 5-6 hours on LOW.

7. Serve warm.

8. Refrigerate or freeze leftovers.

Heavenly Freestyle Pizza Lasagna Roll-Ups

Yield: 8 PIECES

INGREDIENTS:
- 8 uncooked lasagna noodles
- 15 oz. can tomato sauce
- 1 cup pizza sauce
- ½ teaspoon Italian seasoning
- 1 lb. uncooked hot Italian poultry sausage, casings removed if present (I used Wegmans patties, you can use chicken or turkey sausage)
- 2 oz. turkey pepperoni, chopped (reserve 8 slices un-chopped for topping)
- 1 (15 oz.) container fat free Ricotta cheese

- 1 (10 oz.) package frozen chopped spinach, thawed and squeezed until dry
- 1 large egg
- 2 oz. 2% shredded Mozzarella cheese

DIRECTIONS:

6. Pre-heat the oven to 350. Lightly mist a 9×13 baking dish with cooking spray and set aside.

7. Boil and salt a large pot of water and cook lasagna noodles according to package instructions. Drain and rinse with cold water. Lay noodles flat on a clean dry surface and set aside.

8. In a mixing bowl, combine the tomato sauce, pizza sauce and Italian seasoning and stir together. Set aside.

9. Place the sausage in a large skillet over medium heat and cook until browned, breaking the meat up into small pieces as it cooks. When the sausage is cooked through, add the chopped pepperoni and 1/3 cup of the tomato sauce mixture and stir to combine. Remove from heat.

10. In a mixing bowl, combine the ricotta cheese, spinach and egg and stir until well combined. Spoon 1/3 cup of the cheese mixture onto each lasagna noodle and spread across the surface leaving a little room (about ½") at the far end with no toppings. Top the cheese layer on each noodle with the meat mixture from step four, evenly

dividing the meat between the noodles. Starting with one end (not the one with space at the end), roll the noodle over the filling until it becomes a complete roll. Repeat with all noodles.

11. Spoon ½ cup of the tomato sauce mixture into the prepared baking dish and spread across the bottom. Place the lasagna rolls seam down in the dish and spoon or pour the remaining sauce over top. Sprinkle the Mozzarella over the top of the rolls and place a pepperoni on each one. Cover the dish with aluminum foil and bake for 40 minutes.

NUTRITION INFORMATION:

289 calories, 31 g carbs, 9 g sugars, 8 g fat, 2 g saturated fat, 24 g protein, 4 g fiber

Yummy Sea Scallops, Arugula, & Beet Salad

COOKING TIME: 6 -8 minutes

SERVES: 2

INGREDIENTS:

1 tablespoon olive oil,

½ tablespoon red wine vinegar,

1 teaspoon shallot(minced),

½ tablespoon cider vinegar,

¾ tablespoon raw honey,

2.5 ounces baby arugula,

1 cup yellow beets(peeled, diced, cooked),

6 large sea scallops,

Pepper to taste,

Kosher salt to taste,

2 tablespoons goat cheese,

crumbled,

4 grape tomatoes (halved),

and Cooking spray

INSTRUCTIONS:

1) Sprinkle salt and pepper over the scallops. Place a nonstick pan over medium-high heat. Spray with cooking spray. Add scallops. Do not stir and sear until golden brown in color. Flip sides and cook the other side until golden brown. Do not overcook.

2) To make the dressing: Whisk together all the ingredients for the dressing and set aside. Pour dressing over the arugula and toss. Divide the arugula among 2 plates.

3) Top with half the beets, half the tomato, 3 scallops and half the goat cheese over the arugula in the 2 plates.

Serve immediately.

Scrumptious French Onion Soup

COOKING TIME: 35 minutes

SERVES: 3

INGREDIENTS:

1 ½ pounds onions(sliced),

2 teaspoons canola oil,

2 cups beef broth,

2 cups chicken broth,

½ tablespoon all-purpose flour,

½ teaspoon fresh thyme leaves,

2 sprigs fresh thyme,

Salt to taste,

Freshly ground pepper to taste,

3 slices French bread(toasted)

and 1-ounce goat cheese(at room temperature)

INSTRUCTIONS:

1) Place a Dutch oven over medium heat. Add oil. When the oil is heated, add onions and salt and sauté until light brown.

2) Add flour and stir until the flour is light brown. Add thyme sprigs and pepper and stir. Add broth and stir. Lower heat, cover and simmer for about 30 minutes. Discard thyme sprigs.

3) Meanwhile, mix cheese and thyme leaves in a bowl. Spread over the bread slices. Ladle into soup bowls. Serve with a slice of bread each.

Mouthwatering Cheese and Ham Omelet

Ingredients:

½ c. diced ham

¼ c. Parmesan cheese

1/8 tsp. pepper

1/8 tsp. hot pepper sauce

2 Tbsp. green onion, chopped

¼ tsp. salt

2 eggs

4 egg whites

Directions:

1. For this recipe, bring out a bowl and ix together the hot sauce, salt, pepper, eggs, and onion.

2. Take out a skillet and grease it with some cooking spray before heating it up. Pour the mixture into the skillet and let it cook for 5 minutes so it has time to set.

3. Sprinkle the top with the ham and the Parmesan cheese. Fold the omelet in half and let it cook for another minute before serving.

Delicious Oregano Spicy Braised Beef

COOKING TIME: 1 hour

SERVES: 2

INGREDIENTS:

5 cloves garlic,

2 1/2 teaspoons kosher salt,

Black pepper,

1/2 medium onion,

1 lime (juice),

1 tablespoon ground cumin,

1 tablespoon ground oregano,

2 tablespoon chipotles in adobo sauce,

1/2 teaspoon ground cloves,

1 cup water,

3 lbs beef eye of round (all fat trimmed, chopped into 3"
pieces),

1 teaspoon oil

and 3 bay leaves

INSTRUCTIONS:

1) Combine the cloves, water, chipotle, oregano, lime juice,
cumin, onion, and garlic in a blender and blend until smooth.

2) Season the meat with salt and pepper and brown in an
Instant Pot with oil set to the Sauté function. Pour the blended
sauce, and mix in the bay leaves.

3) Select the Manual function for 1 hour at high pressure. Do a
natural release of pressure. Remove the meat and shred it.

4) Mix the shredded meat with 1 ½ cups of the cooking liquid.
Serve and enjoy.

Heavenly Beans & Vegan Nachos In the Pot

Ready in 45 minutes,

5 servings

Ingredients

- 2 cups of dried beans, well rinsed
- 1/2 tablespoon salt
- 5 cloves of garlic, peeled and chopped
- 1 jalapeno - seeded
- 1 diced large onion
- 1 teaspoon paprika
- ½ teaspoon chili powder
- 1 teaspoon cumin
- ½ teaspoon black pepper
- ½ cup salsa
- 4 cups of vegetable broth

Instructions

1. Add all the ingredients into the instant pot and stir well. Tightly close with the lid. Seal the steam valve. Shorten cooking time to about 30 minutes.

2. Leave for at least 10 minutes before releasing the pressure. Open the lid and stir well.

3. Blend the beans to by either mashing in the potato masher, or blending. Drain some of the water off before mashing or blending, and add it back just as you need it to thicken the beans according to preference.

4. Serve warm

Nutrition information
Calories: 613
Carbohydrates: 58.4g
Fats: 32g
Proteins: 25.4g

Irresistible Instant Lemon Garlic Chicken

Ready in 30 minutes,

4 servings

Ingredients

- 2 pounds' chicken breasts
- 1 teaspoon salt
- 1 diced onion
- 1 tablespoon avocado oil or ghee
- 4-5 minced garlic cloves
- 1 cup organic chicken broth
- 1 teaspoon dried parsley
- 1/2 teaspoon paprika
- 1/2cup white cooking wine
- 2 lemons
- 4 teaspoons arrowroot flour

Instructions

1. Set the Instant Pot onto the fry option and add in onion and cooking fat

2. Allow the onions to cook until softened or for 5-10 minutes.

3. Add in the other remaining ingredients with exception of the arrowroot flour and tight lid the pot.

4. Choose the "Poultry" setting and ensure the steam valve is closed. Allow enough time to completely cook, release steam and then carefully remove lid

5. Thicken your sauce by making a slurry by removing some of the sauce from the pot.Add in the arrowroot flour, and reintroduce the slurry into the remaining liquid. Afterwards, stir and serve right.

Nutrition information

Calories: 205.3

Carbohydrates: 1.1g

Fats: 5.8g

Proteins: 35.1g

Yummy Freestyle Corn & Zucchini Summer Frittata

Yield: 6 SLICES

INGREDIENTS:

- 1 medium ear of fresh raw corn
- 1 tablespoon light butter (I use Land O'Lakes)
- 1 cup thin sliced zucchini
- 8 large eggs
- 1/3 cup 2% plain Greek yogurt (I used Fage)
- ¾ teaspoon salt (plus a sprinkle more for the corn & zucchini)
- ¼ teaspoon black pepper (plus a sprinkle more for the corn & zucchini)
- 1 tablespoon diced chives
- ¼ cup sliced fresh basil
- 2 oz. sharp cheddar cheese, shredded (I used Cabot Seriously Sharp)

DIRECTIONS:

1. Pre-heat your oven to 350. Shuck the corn and remove any remaining strings. Use a large sharp knife to cut off the kernels as close to the cob as you can get (I ended up with about 1 cup of kernels).

2. Melt the butter in an 8"-10" *oven-safe* nonstick deep skillet over medium-low heat. Add the corn kernels and the sliced zucchini and stir to coat.

3. Sprinkle with a bit of salt and pepper to taste. Cook, stirring regularly, for 6-8 minutes or until corn and zucchini are cooked through.

4. While the corn and zucchini are cooking, break the eggs into a large mixing bowl and whisk together until just combined.

5. Add the yogurt, salt, black pepper, chives, basil and shredded cheese and stir together until mixed.

6. When the corn and zucchini are cooked, transfer them into the bowl containing the egg mixture and stir together. Spray the skillet you used liberally with cooking spray and then pour the egg mixture into the skillet.

7. Cook on a burner set to medium heat for 5-7 minutes until the very outside edge of the frittata starts to turn opaque/look cooked.

8. Transfer the skillet into the oven and cook for 15-17 minutes until the center is set. Let cool for 5 minutes, then slice into 6 slices and serve.

NUTRITION INFORMATION PER SLICE:

167 calories, 5 g carbs, 2 g sugars, 11 g fat, 5 g saturated fat, 13 g protein, 1 g fiber

Scrumptious Pressure Cooked Chicken Romano

Ready in 25 minutes,

2 servings

Ingredients:

- ½ cup all-purpose flour
- ½ teaspoon salt
- ½ teaspoon pepper
- 6 boneless skinless chicken
- 2 tablespoons oil
- 1 onion minced
- 1 10 ounce can tomato sauce
- 1 teaspoon vinegar
- 1 sliced mushrooms, fresh
- 1 tablespoon sugar
- 1 teaspoon garlic minced
- 1 tablespoon dried oregano
- 1 teaspoon dried basil
- 1 teaspoon of chicken bouillon granules
- 1 cup Romano cheese

Instructions

1. Sauté chicken in oil until golden brown. Add garlic and onion and cook until fragrant or become translucent.

2. Add the remaining ingredients with exception of Romano cheese. Stir well to combine. Secure the Instant Pot lid and set pressure valve to pressure.

3. Select the manual setting and set timer at 10-minutes. When the 10-minutes are up and, allow 10-minutes and then naturally release pressure.

4. Remove the lid, add Romano cheese and stir. Serve over pasta, rice.

Nutrition information

Calories: 108

Carbohydrates: 10g

Fats: 2g

Proteins: 10g

Mouth Watering Spiralized Apple & Cabbage Slaw

COOKING TIME: 5-8 minutes

SERVES: 3

INGREDIENTS:

1 ½ cups red cabbage(shredded),

1 cup green cabbage(shredded),

1 small Granny Smith apple (discard stem),

1 tablespoon golden balsamic vinegar,

1 tablespoon olive oil,

1 teaspoon honey,

¾ teaspoon poppy seeds,

Freshly ground black pepper to taste and Kosher salt to taste

INSTRUCTIONS:

1) Add olive oil, vinegar, poppy seeds, honey, salt, and pepper into a bowl and whisk well.

2) Make noodles of the apple using a spiralizer using a larger blade. Once the noodles are made, cut into smaller pieces using scissors. Place in a bowl.

3) Add cabbage, red as well as white. Pour dressing over it and fold gently until well combined.

Serve as it is or chills and serve later.

Heavenly Freestyle Bean Soup

12 approximately 1 cup servings

Ingredients:

- 2 cans white beans (rinsed and drained)
- 2 cans Lima beans (rinsed and drained)
- 2 cans corn kernels drained
- 1 carton low sodium vegetable broth
- 12 slices Canadian Bacon chopped into small pieces
- Season to taste,

DIRECTIONS:

1. Dump all ingredients into a large crockpot.
2. Stir gently to evenly mix ingredients.
3. Cook on low 6-8 hours.

Delicious Crispy Apple Surprise

Ingredients:

Ground cloves

3 lb. sliced apples

¼ c. sugar

1 tsp. vanilla

¼ tsp. nutmeg

3 Tbsp. butter

1 tsp. water

¼ tsp. cinnamon

Salt

¼ c. brown sugar

½ tsp. ginger

½ c. and 2 Tbsp. flour

½ c. quick cooking oats

Directions;

1. For this recipe, turn on the oven and let it heat up to 375 degrees. Take out a baking dish and cover it with some cooking spray.

2. First we will need to make the topping. To do this, bring out a bowl and combine the oats with the

cinnamon, salt, brown sugar, ginger, and ½ cup of flour.

3. Add in the butter at this time and then place it all into the pastry blender so that you get a nice crumbly mixture. Pour in some water and then press this to make clumps.

4. Now you will want to work on the filling. To do this, bring out a bowl and combine the cloves, sugar, nutmeg, and the rest of the flour. Put in the vanilla and the apples in as well and then pour everything inside a baking dish.

5. Pour your topping over the filling and then place everything into the oven. Bake this all in the oven for 60 minutes.

Heavenly Chicken Taco Soup Recipe

Prep time: 5 mins

Cook time: 30 mins

Total time: 35 mins

Ingredients

- 2 Cups Shredded or Cubed Chicken
- 1 onion, diced
- 1 bell pepper, diced
- 1 poblano pepper, diced
- 2 tomatoes, chopped
- 1 tablespoon garlic, minced
- 6 cups fat free chicken broth
- 1 cup tomato sauce
- 1½ cups kidney beans or pinto beans
- 2 tablespoons taco/fajita seasoning
- 1 tablespoon olive oil

Instructions

1. In a large stockpot, sauté the onion, bell pepper, poblano pepper, and tomato for 5 minutes stirring regularly. You want the vegetables to be tender.
2. Mix in chicken, broth, tomato sauce, garlic, pinto beans, and seasonings.
3. Simmer on medium heat for 30 minutes, stirring occasionally.
4. Serve with preferred garnishes like cheese, sour cream, or tortilla chips.

Tasty Pressure cooked beef ribs

Ready in 25-30 minutes,

2 servings

Ingredients

- 1 rack of beef back ribs
- Dry rub
- ½ cup kosher salt
- ½ cup water
- 4 ounces of applesauce, unsweetened
- 2 tablespoons coconut oil
- 1 teaspoon fish sauce

Instructions

1. Dry the beef back ribs with a paper towel and then, sprinkle with the dry rub and salt. Wrap up in foil and set aside to marinate for two hours.

2. Preheat the broiler, grab the rack from the fridge and cut to fit in the pressure cooker. Put the ribs on a wire rack in a baking sheet rimmed and foil lined.

3. Broil the ribs for 1-2 minutes each side. Add water, fish sauce applesauce and coconut oil to the pressure cooker and stir to combine, add a rack to the pot.

4. Put the ribs into the cooker and tight lid. Bring the heat to high pressure and lower to maintain high pressure. Cook for 20 minutes and release pressure naturally and quickly.

5. Withdraw the ribs and place them back on a wire rack lined with foil and rimmed baking sheet.

6. Simmer the remaining cooking liquid for 5 minutes and skim off any excess fat and adjust seasoning.

7. Coat the racks with the remaining liquid and broil them for one minute.

Nutrition information

Calories: 87

Carbohydrates: 0g

Fats: 7g

Proteins: 4.7g

Yummy Freestyle Fat Free Pimento Chile Chicken

Ingredients:

- 2 ½ c. cooked, chopped chicken breast (chopped into about 1/2" cubes
- ½ c. fat free chicken broth
- 1 ½ c. 98% fat free cream of mushroom soup (I use Campbell's)
- 1 ½ c. Healthy Request Condensed cream of chicken soup
- 1 4-oz. jar pimentos, drained (1/2 c.)
- 2 4-oz. cans Hatch green chiles, chopped and drained (You can add a 3rd can if you're just crazy about chiles like I am.)
- 10 oz. 50% reduced fat sharp cheddar cheese
- 6 oz. of Doritos (by weight) toasted corn tortilla chips, slightly crushed
- Pickled jalapeños, green onions, and/or cherry tomatoes for serving (optional)

Instructions:

1. Mix all ingredients except Doritos and cheese. In a large casserole dish (I use 9" x 13"), layer ½ of chicken mixture, then ½ of cheese, then ½ of the Doritos.

2. Repeat the same layers once more, ending with Doritos on top. Bake at 350° for about 40-45 minutes.

3. Cover top with foil if Doritos begin to brown too much.

4. Serve with pickled jalapeños and/or your favorite salsa.

Delicious Freestyle Ham and Cheese Egg Cups

Yield: 12 EGG CUPS

INGREDIENTS:

- 9 oz. thinly sliced deli ham, divided (I used Hillshire Farm Deli Select)
- 6 large eggs
- 2 egg whites
- ¼ cup skim milk
- ¼ teaspoon salt
- 1/8 teaspoon pepper
- ½ cup chopped fresh spinach leaves
- 2 oz. shredded 2% sharp cheddar cheese, divided

DIRECTIONS:

1. Preheat the oven to 350. Lightly mist 12 cups in a muffin tin with cooking spray. Press a slice of ham into each cup of the muffin tin, arranging the edges to form a ham cup.

2. Chop up the remaining ham (my slices were about ½ ounce each so I had around 3 ounces remaining) and set aside.

3. In a mixing bowl, combine the eggs, egg whites, milk, salt and pepper and whisk together until yolks and whites are fully combined and beaten.

4. Add the reserved chopped ham, the spinach and half of the shredded cheddar and stir together to combine.

5. Spoon the egg mixture evenly into the ham cups and then top each cup with the remaining shredded cheese. Place the tin in the oven and bake for 18-20 minutes until the eggs are set.

NUTRITION INFORMATION PER EGG CUP:
82 calories, 2 g carbs, 1 g sugars, 4 g fat, 2 g saturated fat, 9 g protein, 0 g fiber

Yummy Freestyle Creamy-Tomato-Basil-Soup

Serves: 4

Ingredients

- 1 cup low sodium chicken broth (or vegetable broth if you prefer)
- 1 14 oz. can tomato puree
- 1 cup skim milk
- 4-5 leaves fresh basil
- 3 tsp. olive oil
- 1 stalk celery
- ½ cup onions
- 1 Tbsp. cornstarch
- 1-2 cloves garlic, crushed.
- pepper to taste

Instructions

1. Rough chop onions and celery, transfer them to a food processor or chopper and puree until fine.
2. Heat olive oil in a large pan over medium heat.
3. Add onion and celery mix to pan and sauté until they begin to become translucent.

4. Reduce heat to low and stir in garlic, pepper, chicken stock, and tomato puree, and cornstarch-simmer on low for 5 minutes.
5. Whisk in tomato puree and milk, top with basil leaves, simmer for an additional 10 minutes.
6. Serve topped with a dollop of Greek yogurt or a fresh chopped basil.
7. This makes approximately 4 -1/2 cup servings

Heavenly Low Yolk Egg Salad

COOKING TIME: 5 minutes
SERVES: 4

INGREDIENTS:
8 eggs (hard boiled, peeled),
1 teaspoon Dijon mustard,
8 teaspoons light mayonnaise,
4 tablespoons green scallions or chives,
Freshly ground black pepper and Salt to taste

INSTRUCTIONS:

1) Separate the yolks from the whites. Use only 2 yolks and discard the rest. Chop the 2 yolks and all the whites and place in a bowl.

2) Add rest of the ingredients and fold gently.

Tasty Jerk Turkey Soup

COOKING TIME: 6-7 hours

SERVES: 3

INGREDIENTS:

7.5 ounces canned black beans(drained, rinsed),

7.5 ounces fire roasted diced tomatoes with green chili pepper with its liquid,

½ pound turkey breast(chopped into 1-inch pieces),

1 small onion(chopped),

1 clove garlic(minced),

¼ teaspoon ground ginger,

¼ teaspoon ground allspice,

¼ teaspoon garlic salt, Salt to taste,

¼ teaspoon cayenne pepper,

2 cups chicken broth,

1 tablespoon fresh cilantro(chopped),

and 2 teaspoons fresh lemon juice

INSTRUCTIONS:

1) Mix in a bowl, allspice, cayenne pepper, garlic salt, ginger and a little pepper. Add turkey and toss well. Set aside for a while.

2) Transfer the turkey to a slow cooker. Add remaining ingredients except for lemon juice and cilantro and stir. Cover and cook on 'Low' for 6-7 hours or on 'High' for 2 ½ - 3 hours.

Irresistible Potato and Cheese Casserole

Ingredients:

Salt

Pepper

4 beaten eggs

1 can milk, evaporated

3 oz. bacon, chopped

½ c. scallion, sliced

3 c. potato, shredded

¾ c. cheddar cheese

Directions:

1. For this recipe, turn on the oven and let it heat up to 350 degrees. Take out your baking pan and coat it with some cooking spray.

2. Place the potatoes into the prepared baking pan and then top with some cheese, scallions, and bacon.

3. Now bring out a small bowl and mix together the pepper, salt, eggs, and milk inside. Pour this all on top of the potato mixture.

4. Place this meal inside the oven and let it cook for 40 minutes or until everything has time to set.

5. Take it out of the oven and give it a few minutes to cool down before slicing and enjoying.

Tasty Almond Orange Cornmeal Cake

COOKING TIME: 45 minutes

SERVES: 3

INGREDIENTS:

1 ¼ cups all-purpose flour,

½ cup yellow cornmeal (preferably),

2 teaspoons baking powder,

½ teaspoon salt,

¾ cup plus 1 tablespoon sugar,

½ cup low-fat buttermilk,

1/3 cup olive oil,

2 large eggs,

1 tablespoon grated lemon zest,

2 tablespoons sliced almonds,

2 (1 lb.) containers fresh strawberries (hulled and sliced)

and ¼ cup orange liqueur or orange juice

INSTRUCTIONS:

1) Preheat the oven to 350F. Spray an 8-inch round cake pan with nonstick spray.

2) Combine the flour, cornmeal, baking powder, and salt in a large zip-lock plastic bag; seal bag and mix well. Whisk together ¾ cup of sugar, the buttermilk, oil, eggs, and lemon zest in large bowl.

3) Add flour mixture to buttermilk mixture, stirring just until combined. Pour batter into prepared pan. Scatter almonds over the mixture and sprinkle with remaining 1 tablespoon sugar.

4) Bake until the toothpick inserted into the center of a cake comes out with moist crumbs attached, about 25 -30 minutes. Let cool in the pan on a wire rack for 15 minutes. Remove the cake from the pan and let it cool completely on a rack.

5) Stir together the liqueur and strawberries in a serving bowl. Serve with cake. Enjoy.

Delicious Veggie & Chicken broth

Ready in 45 minutes.

4 servings

Ingredients

- 5 ribs celery
- 1 large onion
- 1 tablespoon apple cider vinegar
- 2 carrots
- 1 frozen or thawed chicken
- 4cloves garlic
- water
- 1tablespoon peppercorns
- 3 tablespoons salt water

Instructions

1. Combine all ingredients in the pressure cooker – cut the vegetables finely.
2. Add water to fill the pressure cooker

3. Cover cooker with lid and pressure gauge on your pressure cooker

4. Cook for 30 minutes while following pressure cooker instructions.

5. Allow cooker to depressurize on its own.

6. Open the cooker carefully and remove the chicken from the broth.

7. Strain the broth to remove veggies and peppercorns.

8. Use the broth for soup and serve.

Nutrition information

Calories: 77

Carbohydrates: 3.4g

Fats: 4.5g

Proteins: 6.6g

Conclusion

Well good job! Well done for completing this book and making it to the conclusion.

As you would now obviously know, so many people worldwide are suffering from health issues and problems, but you won't have to anymore nor should people you care about, as what you have in your hands are the recipes that will allow you to start living the healthy lifestyle you always dreamed of!

As mentioned at the start of the book, the recipes inside this book are incredibly simple! Just by following a few simple guidelines, you will still get to enjoy the kinds of foods you always loved and also achieve your goals!

Last of all, if you found this book useful, make sure to write a great review on the amazon page for the book as that'd be well appreciated!

Good luck on your health and fitness journey!

Made in the USA
Coppell, TX
27 October 2023

23454106R10095